How to Be Dominant in Bed

Even if You Are Anxious or Unconfident

Cheryl Bach

How to Be Dominant in Bed

Publisher: IntimateInk Press

Email: intimateinkpress@gmail.com

This book is a work of nonfiction intended for informational purposes only. The content of this book is based on the author's research, knowledge, and experience, and it is provided with the understanding that the author and publisher are not engaged in rendering legal, medical, or professional advice. The information in this book is not a substitute for professional guidance or assistance. Readers should consult with relevant professionals for advice and assistance regarding their specific situations. The author and publisher disclaim any liability for any loss or risk, personal or otherwise, which is incurred as a consequence, directly or indirectly, of the use and application of any of the contents of this book.

Cover design by IntimateInk Press

Interior layout and design by IntimateInk Press

Printed in USA

Fonts: Google fonts

Image: Freepik.com. This cover has been designed using assets from Freepik.com

For permission to use copyrighted material from this book, please contact the copyright holder listed above.

First Edition: 2024

Distributed by Amazon.com, Inc.

Cheryl Bach

Table of Contents

Introduction

Are you someone who yearns to take control in the bedroom, but struggles with feelings of anxiety or inadequacy? Do you find yourself holding back, afraid of offending your partner or crossing a line you didn't intend to cross? If so, you are not alone, and this book is for you.

In How to Be Dominant in Bed: Even if You Are Anxious or Unconfident, we will explore how to overcome the hurdles that may be holding you back from exploring your dominant side. Whether you are new to BDSM play or simply looking to spice up your sex life, this book will provide you with the guidance, information, and support you need to embrace your dominant desires safely and confidently.

How to Be Dominant in Bed

We will start by defining what dominance means for you and your partner, and examining the importance of consent and communication as cornerstones of a healthy BDSM relationship. From there, we will discuss how to initiate the conversation with your partner about exploring a dominant-submissive dynamic, and how to set the right tone for experimentation.

Throughout the book, we will emphasize the importance of building trust and deepening emotional connection between partners, as well as establishing rules and consistency in your play. We will explore specific techniques and subtle touches that can be used to build anticipation and playfulness, while ensuring that both partners feel safe and respected. And we will delve into the world of bondage and restraints, discussing different types of equipment and techniques, and emphasizing the importance of safety and communication.

At every step, we will address common fears and insecurities that may inhibit your journey toward embracing your dominant side. We will provide practical exercises, tips, and strategies to help you develop self-confidence and technique in a dominant role, while respecting boundaries and consent. We will also examine the ethics and communication necessary to build and maintain a healthy BDSM dynamic, emphasizing the importance of mutual respect, trust, and openness.

Ultimately, this book aims to help you explore your dominant desires in a safe, respectful, and meaningful way, while encouraging you to experiment, expand your repertoire, and keep things fresh. By embracing your dominant side in the bedroom, you can boost confidence in all areas of your life, and deepen emotional connection with your partner in ways that transcend the physical.

How to Be Dominant in Bed

Whether you are new to BDSM play or looking to take your existing dynamic to the next level, How to Be Dominant in Bed: Even if You Are Anxious or Unconfident is the guide you need to overcome your fears and embrace your inner dominant. Let's get started.

Chapter 1

Why Being Dominant in Bed Can Be Sexy and Exciting

Dominance can be an incredibly attractive quality in any context, but particularly so in the bedroom. Whether you're looking to spice up a long-term relationship, trying something new with a casual fling, or simply exploring your own desires, embracing your dominant side in bed can bring some serious heat to your sex life.

In this chapter, we will explore some of the reasons why being dominant in bed can be so sexy and exciting. From the thrill of control to the heightened emotional connection, we will examine the many benefits of dominant play, and how it can enhance your overall sexual experience.

How to Be Dominant in Bed

Firstly, dominance allows for a heightened sense of control. When you are the dominant partner in bed, you are able to take charge and dictate the pace, rhythm, and intensity of the experience. This can be incredibly thrilling and empowering, allowing you to feel a sense of agency and mastery over the situation. It can also create an atmosphere of anticipation and excitement, as your partner waits to see what you will do next and how they will respond.

Being dominant in bed can also deepen the emotional connection between partners. Creating an unequal power dynamic, with one partner assuming the role of authority, can foster a greater sense of intimacy and trust between both individuals. By opening up and exploring your desires and fantasies with your partner, you lay the groundwork for a stronger and more communicative relationship.

On top of that, being dominant can simply be incredibly sexy. The confidence and assertiveness required to take on this role can be intoxicating, both for you and your partner. As you tease and play with your partner, pushing them to their limits and perhaps even revealing new aspects of their own desires, the boundaries between you both start to blur. The blurred lines can create a sense of escape from everyday life and into a world of passion and excitement, accentuating raw emotions while elevating attraction and chemistry between partners.

Dominance can also be an opportunity for creative play and experimentation. As the dominant partner, you have a license to explore new techniques and ideas that might not be on your partner's radar. This can lead to new and exciting sexual experiences that go beyond the usual comfort zones, making the sex feel fresh, spontaneous and thrilling each time.

How to Be Dominant in Bed

In conclusion, embracing your dominant side in bed can lead to a range of exciting sexual experiences, with rewards that can cascade beyond the bedroom to enhance the confidence, intimacy, and creativity in your relationship. The power, control and excitement created by taking charge ramps up the energy and give a new meaning to adventurous sex while also deepening the emotional connection between partners. When done with consent and healthy communication, dominant behavior in bed can be incredibly sexy and exciting, leading to an exploration of new fantasies and desires that otherwise may not have been explored. It is important to remember that being dominant doesn't necessarily mean being aggressive or disrespectful. Instead, it is about creating a safe space where both partners feel comfortable exploring their vulnerabilities, desires, and pleasures.

In the following chapters, we will dive deeper into the various aspects of dominant behavior in bed, from building trust through clear communication, to how to initiate the conversation with your partner, and specific tips and techniques to enhance the power dynamic between you and your partner. With the right mindset and tools, anyone can confidently embrace their dominance in bed, take control, and elevate their sexual experiences to a new level of intimacy and excitement.

So, if you're ready to explore the sexy and exciting world of dominant behavior in bed, let's do it together. In the upcoming chapters of this book, we will show you how to tap into your dominant side and bring that energy into your sexual encounters, even if you are anxious or unconfident.

Through a combination of practical advice, personal anecdotes, and real-life scenarios, we will help you cultivate the confidence and skills needed to become a strong and effective dominant partner.

How to Be Dominant in Bed

So what are you waiting for? Let's dive into the world of dominant behavior and unleash a new level of sexual excitement and thrill!

Chapter 2

Understanding What Dominance Means for You and Your Partner

Dominance can mean different things to different people, and it's essential to understand what it means for you and your partner before you start exploring it in bed. Knowing how you both feel about dominance and power dynamics will help you establish consensual and enjoyable aspects of the role-play without hurting your partner.

In this chapter, we explore what it means to be dominant in bed, how it can impact you and your partner, and the importance of discussing your desires explicitly with each other.

How to Be Dominant in Bed

Firstly, being dominant is a behavior that involves the willingness and ability to take on a more assertive role in sexual encounters. Dominance doesn't necessarily mean one person is superior or inferior; it's just about controlling the dynamic between you and your partner, which often can be the source of heightened satisfaction.

While dominance can be exciting and liberating for some people, it's important to understand that it may not be everyone's cup of tea. The first step in exploring your dominant side is to have honest and open communication with your partner and determine if they are interested in exploring this dynamic as well. If you're already in a relationship, it may be easier to bring up the topic, but if you're single, it's important to discuss boundaries and desires explicitly before engaging in any sexual activity.

Once you both have established consent and interest, understanding your motivations for exploring dominance in bed is crucial. Are you looking to explore new kinks, experiment with power dynamics, or simply trying something fun? Knowing what you want from your dominant side can help you communicate better with your partner and create something fulfilling for you both.

It's essential to keep in mind that dominance doesn't necessarily mean being aggressive or disrespectful to your partner. It also doesn't have to be a 24/7 lifestyle or something you both engage in every time you have sex. Dominance can be as simple as taking control during foreplay, giving commands, or trying out a particular sexual position. It's entirely adaptable to your preferences.

For some people, dominance may be tied to feelings of power, control, and even sadism, while others may embrace it as a way to explore vulnerability, submissiveness, and pleasure. Understanding your motivations for exploring

How to Be Dominant in Bed

dominance will help you approach the role more authentically and confidently.

Once you both have established consent, interests, and motivations, it's essential to discuss boundaries around what is and isn't okay, and any relevant safe words or signals for when things need to slow down or stop. Consent and communication are pivotal in making sure that dominance in the bedroom is enjoyable and respectful for both partners.

Another critical aspect of understanding dominance is understanding that it's not one size fits all. Different people have different preferences when it comes to power dynamics and control, and exploring what works for you and your partner on a case-by-case basis is essential.

One partner may enjoy being assertive and giving commands, while the other may enjoy being submissive and following those commands. The key is finding a balance that works for both partners and establishing boundaries that keep everyone comfortable and safe.

In conclusion, exploring dominance in bed can be an exciting and satisfying part of your sexual repertoire. However, it's important to understand what it means to you and your partner, communicate openly and honestly about your interests and boundaries, and approach the role with empathy, authenticity, and respect. With these principles in mind, exploring dominance will be a rewarding experience that can deepen your connection and bring new levels of pleasure and satisfaction to your sexual encounters.

Remember to maintain open and consistent communication with your partner and be vigilant in checking in with each other throughout the experience to ensure that boundaries and emotional well-being are being respected. Don't hesitate to adjust or pause the role-play if either partner feels uncomfortable or unsafe.

In summary, dominance in bed can mean a variety of things, and it's up to you and your partner to explore what works best for your relationship dynamic. With open communication, clear consent, and mutual respect, exploring dominance can be liberating, empowering, and enjoyable for you and your partner alike.

Chapter 3

Creating a Dom/Sub Dynamic

The Dom/Sub or dominant/submissive dynamic is an aspect of the BDSM world that focuses on power imbalances within a sexual relationship. In this chapter, we will explore how you can create a Dom/Sub dynamic in the bedroom, starting with the conversation and setting the tone.

Starting the Conversation

Initially, introducing the idea of a Dom/Sub relationship to your partner can be nerve-racking and scary. Many people fear that they may be judged or rejected if they express their desire for this lifestyle. However, the best way to set up this type of play is through open and honest communication.

How to Be Dominant in Bed

Start by explaining why you feel it's important to you personally and what draws you to a dominant role in the bedroom. Be honest and authentic, but also empathetic to your partner's potential fears or concerns. Remember that it's essential to have this conversation in a non-judgmental, safe, and open environment, and be willing to listen to and consider your partner's feelings.

Setting the Tone

Once you have established the desire to explore Dom/Sub dynamics, it's crucial to discuss boundaries and set expectations with your partner. Setting boundaries will help you keep your partner safe physically and emotionally and will define what is acceptable within this role-play.

It's important to establish a safe word or signal, an easy and safe way for your partner to indicate if they are feeling uncomfortable or want to slow down or stop altogether. This way, you can immediately respond to their needs and make sure the experience remains comfortable and enjoyable for both of you.

Another way to help set the tone is to agree on the specific language that will be used in the Dom/Sub dynamic. This can include titles such as "Master" or "Mistress," specific words or phrases that signify commands or requests, or even limitations on the kind of language that is permitted. It's important to remember that while exploring this dynamic, both partners must be willing and enthusiastic, and neither should feel pressured to engage in something that causes discomfort.

As the dominant partner, it's essential to convey confidence in your role. This doesn't mean being overly aggressive or disrespectful to your partner; instead, it involves an underlying sense of authority, self-assurance, and a willingness to take a leadership role in the relationship. This can be achieved through establishing and maintaining eye contact, speaking with firmness and clarity, and using body language to indicate your dominance.

For the submissive partner, it's equally important to be comfortable communicating boundaries and needs openly and honestly. This could include discussing limitations on certain acts, clarifying the level of pain or discomfort that is acceptable, or requesting breaks or pauses if needed. It is crucial to establish a sense of trust between partners – the submissive partner must feel safe and protected while being in a vulnerable position.

Finally, it's worth emphasizing that the Dom/Sub dynamic is a shared endeavor that both partners must be committed to maintaining. As the dominant partner, you must work closely with your partner to ensure that you understand and respect their boundaries while still maintaining the desired power dynamic. Being attentive to your partner's needs and giving them space to communicate their desires will ensure that the experience is satisfying and rewarding for both parties.

In conclusion, creating a Dom/Sub dynamic requires an open, honest dialogue between partners. This discussion should include establishing clear boundaries, setting expectations, and agreeing on the language and behaviors that will be used within the dynamic. As the dominant partner, you should aim to convey confidence through your speech and body language, while staying attentive and respectful of your partner's needs throughout the experience. Similarly, as the submissive partner, you must communicate your boundaries and comfort levels clearly, ensuring that you feel safe and protected at all times. By establishing a safe, open, and trusting environment, both partners can find pleasure and fulfillment in the Dom/Sub dynamic.

How to Be Dominant in Bed

Chapter 4

Finding and Exploring Your Dominance

Dominance, especially in the bedroom, comes naturally to some people. However, for others, it can be a learned skill that requires practice and confidence building. In this chapter, we will discuss how to find and explore your dominant side, develop your confidence, and hone your technique.

Understanding Dominant Qualities

Before developing your dominance, it's vital to understand what qualities define a dominant partner. Domination isn't about being aggressive or controlling, but rather displaying qualities that indicate leadership and authority. Some common dominant traits include:

Confidence: It's essential to exude confidence in your role as the dominant partner, which is achieved through a deep understanding of your desires and your partner's boundaries, as well as clear communication and an attitude of assertiveness in bed.

Control: As the dominant partner, you must take control of the situation and set the tone for the experience. It's crucial to establish boundaries, set expectations, and lead your partner with confidence, being comfortable making decisions and leading.

Assertiveness: It's important to be assertive in your communication with your partner, giving clear commands and being willing to guide them throughout the experience. This doesn't involve being rude or disrespectful but rather

Cheryl Bach

demonstrating an underlying sense of authority and leadership.

Sensuality: Domination can still be sensual and intimate, even with a power dynamic between partners. Being in control means being attentive to your partner's needs and desires, creating a pleasurable experience for both parties.

Finding Your Dominant Side

To find and explore your dominant side, it's essential to understand your own desires, needs, and boundaries. Take time to reflect on what you find sexy and erotic, and what scenarios turn you on. Think about what aspects of being the dominant partner appeal to you, and what kind of power dynamic you would like to explore with your partner.

It's also important to communicate openly and honestly with your partner. Discuss your desires and boundaries with them and make sure they are comfortable and on board with the power dynamic you want to explore together. Establishing clear communication and understanding each other's needs will help create a safe and fulfilling experience for both partners.

Building Confidence

Confidence is key to being a successful dominant partner, but it's not something that comes naturally to everyone. If you're feeling anxious or insecure about taking on a dominant role, there are several techniques you can use to build confidence.

One way to boost confidence is through knowledge. Take the time to research different power dynamic scenarios and techniques, and practice them in your mind or on your own before trying them in the bedroom. This will give you a sense of what works for you and what doesn't, and help you feel more prepared when the time comes to take on a dominant role.

Another way to build confidence is through physical exercise and body language. Exercise can help increase feelings of power and control, while adopting a confident posture (such as standing tall with shoulders back) can help convey a dominant presence.

Practicing Technique

Once you have a clear understanding of what it means to be a dominant partner and have built up your confidence, it's time to start practicing technique. There are several techniques you can use to assert your dominance, including:

Giving commands: As the dominant partner, you are the one in control, so don't be afraid to give commands to guide your partner throughout the experience.

How to Be Dominant in Bed

Using physical restraints: If you and your partner are comfortable with it, physical restraints such as handcuffs or ropes can help establish a power dynamic. However, it's important to communicate clearly about boundaries and safety before using any kind of restraint.

Spanking or other forms of impact play: Impact play is when one partner strikes the other for erotic purposes. This can be achieved through spanking, slapping, or other techniques. As always, clear communication and boundaries are essential.

Dirty talk: Using dominant language and dirty talk can help establish a power dynamic and make the submissive partner feel more controlled.

In conclusion, developing your dominance takes time and practice, but with clear communication, confidence building, and technique development, you can become a successful dominant partner in the bedroom. Remember to approach the power dynamic with respect and understanding for your partner's needs and boundaries, while staying true to your own desires and preferences. By exploring your dominant side and taking the time to understand yourself and your partner, you can create a safe and fulfilling experience for both parties. Have fun and remember to prioritize communication, respect, and consent in all aspects of your sexual experiences.

How to Be Dominant in Bed

Cheryl Bach

Chapter 5

Techniques and Subtle Touches

Being dominant in bed isn't just about taking control, it's also about building anticipation, creating a sense of playfulness, and using subtle touches to enhance the experience. In this chapter, we will discuss how techniques like teasing, anticipation, and subtle touches can work to build anticipation and create a memorable sexual experience for both partners.

Teasing and Anticipation

One of the most powerful techniques for building anticipation is teasing. Starting slowly and building up to the main event can help make the sexual experience more intense and enjoyable for both parties.

To start, try starting with light touches or kisses, then gradually building up the intensity. This can include circling your partner's sensitive areas with your fingers or tongue, playing with their hair, or whispering dirty talk in their ear, all while building up the anticipation.

Another great way to build anticipation is to use teasing and delay tactics. This can involve stopping the action just when it's getting good, then pulling back and delaying gratification for a bit. This can be achieved by changing things up mid-act, moving your attention to other areas of the body, or simply switching the pace and rhythm of your movements.

By using these methods to tease your partner, you can create a sense of anticipation and excitement that will make the final release even more intense and satisfying.

Cheryl Bach

Subtle Touches

Using subtle touches and gestures can also help build anticipation and create a playful atmosphere during sexual activities. This can include things like tickling, playfully biting, or lightly scratching your partner in a teasing manner.

It's important to remember that communication plays a critical role in these types of touches. Before incorporating them into your sexual activities, make sure you have discussed them with your partner and received their consent. Some people may not enjoy tickling or biting, so it's important to respect each other's boundaries and preferences.

Other ways to use subtle touches include incorporating toys into your play (such as feathers or a vibrator), rubbing your body against your partner's, or simply touching your partner in unexpected and playful ways.

How to Be Dominant in Bed

Incorporating these methods to create a more playful and fun atmosphere during sex can help both partners relax and enjoy the experience. By using teasing and delay tactics, building anticipation, and incorporating subtle touches and gestures, you can create a memorable sexual experience that both you and your partner will cherish.

In conclusion, being dominant in bed doesn't have to be all about power and control. By using techniques like teasing, building anticipation, and incorporating subtle touches and gestures, you can add playfulness into your Dom/Sub Dynamic and make your bedroom activities a little more exciting. However, it's important to remember that communication and consent are essential in all aspects of sexual activity.

As the dominant partner, it's your responsibility to listen to your partner's needs and boundaries and respect them. By doing so, you can build trust and establish a safe and enjoyable environment for both parties. With these techniques and a focus on communication and consent, you can become a confident and successful dominant partner in the bedroom.

How to Be Dominant in Bed

Chapter 6

Bondage and Restraints

Bondage and restraint play can be an exciting way to explore your dominant role in the bedroom. However, it's important to understand the risks involved and take steps to ensure that both you and your partner are safe and comfortable. In this chapter, we will discuss how to incorporate bondage and restraints into your sexual activities while staying safe and respecting each other's boundaries.

Understanding the Risks of Bondage and Restraint Play

Before incorporating bondage or restraints into your sexual activities, it is important to understand the potential risks. One of the main risks of bondage and restraint play is the possibility of injury. This can occur if restraints are too tight, if the submissive partner experiences circulation problems, or if they struggle too much against the restraints.

Another risk is emotional discomfort or distress. Bondage and restraint play can be especially intense, and it's important to consider the emotional impact of engaging in these activities. Some people may experience anxiety or fear during bondage or restraint play, and it's important to have clear communication and establish safe words or signals in case things get too intense.

Knowing Your Limits and Establishing Boundaries

As with any sexual activity, it's important to communicate and establish boundaries before engaging in bondage or restraint play. This includes discussing your limits, what is and isn't okay, and what measures you will take to ensure safety.

Before using restraints, it's also important to consider factors like the submissive partner's physical limitations and any medical conditions that could be exacerbated by the use of restraints.

Choosing the Right Restraints

When choosing restraints, it's important to select materials that are safe and comfortable for both you and your partner. Some common types of restraints used in bondage play include handcuffs, rope, and bondage tape.

If you're using handcuffs, make sure they are specially designed for use during sex and are not too tight or uncomfortable. Rope should be soft and smooth to prevent rope burn or irritation. When using bondage tape, make sure you don't wrap it too tightly around an area as it can cut off circulation.

It's also important to choose restraints that can be easily removed in case of an emergency. Always have a pair of safety scissors on hand in case you need to quickly release your partner from the restraints.

Safe Words and Signals

Establishing safe words or signals is crucial during bondage and restraint play. A safe word is a word agreed upon by both partners that signals the need to stop or slow down. Safe signals can also be used if a partner's mouth is gagged or if verbal communication isn't possible.

When choosing a safe word or signal, avoid using words or actions that could be easily confused with common sounds or actions during sex. Some popular safe words include "red," "yellow," and "green."

It's important to remember that when a safe word or signal is used, play should stop immediately to allow for communication and to ensure both partners' safety and comfort.

Communicating Throughout the Play

During bondage and restraint play, communication is key. As the dominant partner, it's important to frequently check in with your submissive partner and ask how they're feeling. You can also use non-verbal cues, such as checking their body language or facial expressions, to gauge their comfort level.

If your partner seems uncomfortable or distressed, don't be afraid to stop the play and address any concerns.

How to Be Dominant in Bed

Taking Care of Your Partner's Needs

As the dominant partner, it's your responsibility to take care of your partner's needs during bondage and restraint play. This includes ensuring that they have a safe and comfortable position, providing water or snacks if needed, and checking on their physical and emotional well-being throughout the play.

Aftercare is also an important part of taking care of your partner's needs. After bondage and restraint play, it's common for the submissive partner to experience strong emotions, including feelings of vulnerability, sadness, or even guilt. As the dominant partner, it's important to be there for your partner during this time and provide comfort and reassurance.

In conclusion, bondage and restraint play can be an exciting way to explore your dominant side in the bedroom. However, it's important to approach these activities with caution and respect for both you and your partner's boundaries and safety. Remember to establish clear communication, know your limits, choose the right restraints, use safe words or signals, communicate throughout the play, and take care of your partner's needs, including providing aftercare.

By incorporating these safety measures into your bondage and restraint play, you can experience all the excitement and pleasure that come with exploring your dominant side while keeping both you and your partner safe and comfortable. As with any sexual activity, always prioritize consent and respect for your partner's boundaries and emotions.

How to Be Dominant in Bed

Chapter 7

Punishment and Reward

Punishment and reward play an important role when it comes to being dominant in bed. It helps to establish rules and consistency in your relationship, making it easier for both you and your partner to explore your sexual desires. In this chapter, we'll discuss how to establish rules, create a system of punishment and reward, and maintain consistency in your role as a dominant partner.

Establishing Rules

Establishing rules is an essential part of being a dominant partner. These rules can be specific, such as limiting physical touch during certain times, or general, such as obeying commands and following instructions. When establishing rules, it's important to have a clear understanding of what you and your partner expect from the relationship.

It's important to communicate openly with your partner about their limits and boundaries. They should feel comfortable expressing their boundaries with you without fear of judgment or backlash.

When establishing rules, it's important to make sure they're reasonable and achievable. It's also important to remember that rules are not set in stone, and they can be amended or changed as needed. Be open to feedback from your partner and be willing to adjust the rules accordingly.

Creating a System of Punishment and Reward

Once rules have been established, it's important to create a system of punishment and reward. Punishment can be used to reinforce the rules and boundaries that have been established. It should be proportional to the offense committed and should be fair and consistent.

Rewards, on the other hand, can be used to incentivize good behavior and reinforce positive actions. They can be as simple as praise or as elaborate as a special treat or activity for your partner.

It's important to communicate the punishment and reward system with your partner to ensure that they're aware of the consequences of breaking the rules and the benefits of following them. It's important to note that punishment and reward should not be used to manipulate or control your partner, but to reinforce a healthy and fulfilling relationship.

Maintaining Consistency

Consistency is key when it comes to being a dominant partner. Once rules have been established and a system of punishment and reward has been created, it's important to maintain consistency in enforcing them.

Inconsistency can lead to confusion and frustration on both you and your partner's parts. It's important to consistently enforce the rules while also being fair and attentive to your partner's needs.

In conclusion, in order to be a confident and successful dominant partner, it's important to establish clear rules, create a system of punishment and reward, and maintain consistency in enforcing them. Remember that communication is the foundation of a healthy, fulfilling sexual relationship. Make sure you and your partner are on the same page about their boundaries, and always listen to their feedback and adjust accordingly. By incorporating punishment and reward, you can make your sexual experiences more exciting and add an element of structure and discipline to your sex life.

As a dominant partner, it's important to remember to prioritize your partner's well-being and happiness. Your goal is not to control or manipulate them but to enhance your shared sexual experiences and foster a fulfilling and positive relationship.

By following these guidelines for establishing rules, creating a system of punishment and reward, and maintaining consistency, you can become a confident and successful dominant partner in the bedroom.

How to Be Dominant in Bed

Chapter 8

Do's and Don'ts

Being a dominant partner requires the ability to communicate effectively and ethically with your submissive partner. In this chapter, we'll explore the do's and don'ts of communication and ethics to deepen emotional connection during sex.

Do's

Establish Clear Communication

Effective communication is the foundation of any good sexual relationship, especially in BDSM. You must establish clear communication channels with your partner and listen to their feedback, desires, and boundaries to become a confident and successful dominant partner.

How to Be Dominant in Bed

Prioritize Consent

Consent is essential in BDSM play. Before engaging in any activities, ensure that you and your partner have discussed the boundaries, and agree on them. Respect their limits and never push them beyond their comfort zone.

Respect Your Partner

Respect is critical in any relationship, including BDSM ones. Show your partner that you care for them and their well-being by respecting their boundaries and listening to their needs.

Prioritize Emotional Connection

Deepening emotional connection with your partner is an essential part of being a dominant partner. Show your partner that you care about them and their needs, not just in a physical sense but in an emotional one as well.

Cheryl Bach

Create a Safe Space

Creating a safe space is essential in BDSM play. Your partner should feel safe physically and emotionally during all aspects of your sexual relationship.

Don'ts

Don't Compromise on Consent

Consent is non-negotiable in BDSM. If your partner does not give their consent for certain activities, do not try to push them beyond their comfort zone.

Don't Disrespect Boundaries

Respect your partner's boundaries and limits. Never try to pressure or coerce them into anything they are uncomfortable with.

How to Be Dominant in Bed

Don't Make Assumptions

Don't assume that your partner will be okay with certain activities just because they have engaged in them before. Always discuss and confirm activities before engaging in them to ensure everyone is comfortable and enthusiastic.

Don't Disregard Your Partner's Emotions

Your partner's emotional well-being is just as important as their physical safety. Don't disregard their emotions or push them beyond their emotional limits.

Don't Be Judgmental

As a dominant partner, it's important to prioritize acceptance and non-judgmental behavior towards your partner. Avoid shaming or judging them for their interests or desires.

Cheryl Bach

Communication Strategies

Active Listening

Active listening involves paying close attention to what your partner is saying, both verbally and non-verbally. When they are communicating their desires, boundaries, and feedback to you, make sure to listen attentively and respond in an understanding and respectful manner.

Use Empathetic Language

Using empathetic language involves speaking in a way that shows you understand and care about your partner's feelings. Use phrases like "I understand how you feel" or "I can see why that would be important to you" to show your partner that you are listening and empathizing with them.

Check-In Regularly

Check-ins are essential in maintaining emotional connection and ensuring that both you and your partner are comfortable

How to Be Dominant in Bed

during sex. Check-in regularly with your partner throughout the session to get feedback and ensure that they are still comfortable with the activities you are engaging in.

Use Safe Words

Safe words are essential in BDSM play. They provide a way for your partner to communicate when they are uncomfortable or need a break. Agree on a safe word before beginning any activities, and make sure to respect it if your partner uses it during play.

Use Positive Reinforcement

Positive reinforcement involves providing rewards for good behavior. When your partner follows your rules and boundaries or engages in activities that you both enjoy, provide positive feedback to reinforce their behavior and encourage them to continue.

In conclusion, being a dominant partner requires responsible and ethical communication strategies that prioritize both partners' well-being and emotional connection. By prioritizing clear communication, respect for boundaries and emotions, and building an open and accepting communication channel through strategies like active listening, empathetic language, regular check-ins, safe words, and positive reinforcement, you can deepen your emotional connection and create fulfilling sexual experiences for both you and your partner.

How to Be Dominant in Bed

Chapter 9

Experimentation and Exploration

If you want to be a dominant lover, the last thing you want is to get stuck in a rut. It's important to constantly expand your repertoire of sexual activities and experiment with new ways of pleasuring your partner.

One way to keep things fresh is to try out different positions. Don't just stick to the tried-and-true missionary position. Mix it up with some doggy-style, cowgirl or even standing positions. Not only will this variety keep things exciting for both of you, but it will also give you a chance to assert your dominance in different ways.

How to Be Dominant in Bed

Another way to experiment and explore is to incorporate different toys and tools into your sex life. You don't have to be all about whips and chains, but even something as simple as a blindfold or handcuffs can add a new dimension to your lovemaking. Plus, using toys or props can be a great way to assert your dominance in a safe and consensual way.

When it comes to being dominant, words can be incredibly powerful. Don't be afraid to talk dirty to your partner and use your voice to command and control them in the bedroom. But always make sure to pay attention to their responses and adjust accordingly - you never want to push someone too far or cross any boundaries.

Most importantly, remember that communication is key. Don't be afraid to ask your partner what they like and what they're interested in trying. By openly discussing your desires and fantasies, you can work together to expand your sexual repertoire and keep things fresh and exciting.

Ultimately, being a dominant lover is all about creating an atmosphere of trust and consent, where both partners feel comfortable exploring their desires and pushing their boundaries.

Lastly, don't forget to prioritize your own pleasure as well. Being dominant doesn't mean you should only focus on your partner's pleasure. It's important for both of you to enjoy yourselves and for you to feel confident and fulfilled as a lover.

To sum it up, if you want to be dominant in bed, experimentation and exploration are key. Try new positions, incorporate toys and props, communicate openly with your partner and prioritize your own pleasure. With a little confidence and creativity, you can keep your sex life fresh and exciting, while also asserting your dominance in safe and consensual ways.

How to Be Dominant in Bed

Conclusion

In conclusion, being dominant in bed is not about being controlling or abusive towards your partner. Rather, it's about creating a consensual and trusting environment where you can explore your desires and assert your dominance in a safe and healthy way.

Throughout this book, we've covered a range of topics, from building confidence and overcoming anxiety in the bedroom, to exploring different positions and incorporating toys and props. But at the heart of it all, what's most important is communication.

By talking openly with your partner about your desires and boundaries, you can create a space where you both feel comfortable exploring new avenues of pleasure and desire. And by prioritizing each other's pleasure and well-being, you can ensure that your sexual experiences are fulfilling, rewarding, and empowering for both you and your partner.

Remember that being dominant can take many different forms - it's not just about being forceful or demanding. Some people may find that their dominance is more subtle, with a focus on taking control and setting the pace during sex. Others may prefer to engage in role play or BDSM activities that more explicitly involve power dynamics.

Despite these differences, the most important thing is to always prioritize communication, consent, and mutual pleasure and well-being. With these things at the forefront of your mind, you can confidently explore your dominant side and enjoy a fulfilling and exciting sex life with your partner.

Cheryl Bach

Thank you for reading "How to Be Dominant in Bed: Even if You Are Anxious or Unconfident." I hope this book has been helpful in empowering you to explore your desires and assert your dominance in a healthy and consensual way. Remember to celebrate your sexuality and never be ashamed of what you enjoy in the bedroom. With an open mind and a willingness to communicate, you can build a fulfilling and lasting sexual relationship with your partner.

So go forth, experiment, and don't be afraid to take control. You have the power to be an amazing lover and to experience great pleasure and satisfaction with your partner. I wish you all the best on your journey towards sexual dominance!

How to Be Dominant in Bed

www.ingramcontent.com/pod-product-compliance
Lightning Source LLC
Chambersburg PA
CBHW051655250726
48653CB00007B/2684